STICKING TO YOUR PREGNANCY PLAN

Dr. Talya Miron-Shatz and the Buddy&Soul team

INTRODUCTION: WELCOME TO STICKING TO YOUR PREGNANCY PLAN

You're having a baby (yay!) and you want everything to go smoothly. Following your doctor's orders concerning medication, vitamins, lifestyle changes, and diet is an important part of the plan...but that sure as heck ain't to say it's easy.

This book offers you a fresh new look at sticking to your medical provider's prenatal "rules." We'll explore the cognitive, emotional, and behavioral elements that can help you improve your health outcomes, and of course, your baby's.

There are three goals that we had in mind while creating this book. We want you to:

- Assume responsibility for sticking to your pregnancy health regimen.
- Delve deeply into what may be holding you back from properly adhering to a healthy pregnant lifestyle.
- Implement practical, research-based tools to help improve your adherence to your pregnancy plan.

In order to ensure the best possible health outcomes, your medical provider has likely set a few requirements for you. You might be taking folic acid and a prenatal supplement. Perhaps you need iron as well, or other medications or hormones to help maintain your pregnancy. Then, of course, there are those pesky dietary requirements like no raw fish or alcohol and highly limited caffeine, to name a few. And, if you've developed gestational diabetes, preeclampsia, or some other 'fun' pregnancy condition, you might have even more restrictions on top of all that.

On one hand, it can be overwhelming to think of all the lifestyle changes you're expected to make. How are you going to maintain these new routines, especially when every part of you aches and your hormones are more active than Jane Fonda in the 1980s? On the other hand, you know that you are not the only one impacted by the choices you make right now. You and your baby are in this together.

That's where Buddy&Soul comes in. We trust that for the most part you know the importance of sticking to recommended pregnancy guidelines and lifestyle changes and you really want to follow through. But there might still be a gap. If this is the first time in a decade you've been required to trade in your nightly glass of wine for some sparkling water, then yes, it will be an adjustment.

This book will enable you to close the gap and stay on top of your health game. You'll learn to take ownership of your prenatal health decisions, delve deeply into what gets in your way, and practice research-based strategies to help optimize your adherence.

Because doing what's best for you and your baby is what it's all about.

INTRODUCTION: Welcome to Sticking to Your Pregnancy Plan .... Page 2

How to Use This Book .... Page 4

Why I Created Buddy&Soul .... Page 5

STRATEGY 1: Begin with the end in mind .... Page 7

STRATEGY 2: Engage the power of your thoughts .... Page 15

STRATEGY 3: Up your knowledge base .... Page 22

STRATEGY 4: Adjust your expectations .... Page 29

STRATEGY 5: Identify your prenatal adherence hurdles .... Page 36

STRATEGY 6: Get some support .... Page 44

STRATEGY 7: Rate your conscientiousness level .... Page 51

STRATEGY 8: Make it a habit .... Page 59

STRATEGY 9: Make a pregnancy rule .... Page 66

STRATEGY 10: Celebrate your self-control .... Page 73

Where Do We Go From Here.. Page 81

In this book you'll find ten great strategies for achieving the goals we listed above. You'll also find inspiring content and exercises you can engage with to help you stick to your pregnancy plan.

You will get the most out of this book by going through the strategies and associated exercises one by one. Of course, you can also simply read it the whole way through. But we recommend using this book by going through it in order, watching the TED talks, and doing the exercises. We have found the best way to do the exercises is by dedicating a notebook as your course journal. If you're reading this book on a PC, feel free to create a text file and use that as your course journal. Or you could simply use a good ol' pen and paper to do the exercises. Either way, we recommend keeping some method of writing handy while you go through the exercises in this book to optimize what you get out of it.

To maximize your experience with the Buddy and Soul book, share your thoughts and insights with us on social media! Post pictures relating to your progress on Instagram and Twitter, tagging @Buddy_N_Soul, and Facebook @Buddy&Soul.   By sharing with us on social media, not only can you help others with their personal journeys, you can read about those facing similar challenges.

Direct message us YOUR story @Buddy_N_Soul on Instagram and be anonymously featured for a chance to **win a Buddy&Soul three month free membership**.

If you really want to go all the way, visit our website, BuddynSoul.com, and explore all that we have to offer beyond 'Sticking to Your Pregnancy Plan'. In fact, we have three other books in the Pregnancy series that we think you might benefit from: Relationship Saver During Pregnancy, Loving Your Pregnant Body, and Acing the Fourth Trimester.

I'm Dr. Talya Miron-Shatz, CEO of Buddy&Soul, where Sticking to Your Pregnancy Plan and many more e-courses and books come from. I have a PhD in psychology and was very fortunate to do my post-doc at Princeton University with Nobel Laureate Daniel Kahneman. I've also taught at the Wharton Business School, University of Pennsylvania. Now I'm a professor at the Ono Academic College, and a visiting researcher at Cambridge University. I used to study happiness, and for a long time now, I've been studying medical decision making and helping organizations support people on their way to joy and health. One thing

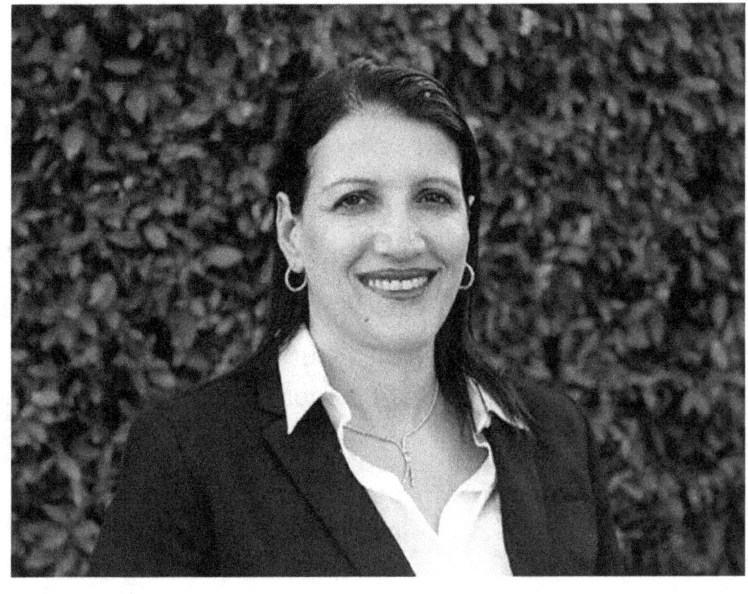

that struck me as unfair was that we were expecting people to change their life for good but weren't giving them the tools to do so. People deserve all the help they can get when breaking out of old patterns and moving their lives forward.

This is what Buddy&Soul does.

We support you in many ways by providing science-based actionable ways to sustain your body and mind. We help you sleep better, spark a change in your eating habits, and manage stress. We teach you how to create new habits and how to engage your willpower. We help you grow, claim your self-esteem, cultivate authenticity, reframe your life story, achieve your goals and so much more. Including Sticking to Your Pregnancy Plan.

We created unique course clusters for people dealing with specific challenges: students, patients, and pregnant women.

Everything you need to change your life for good.

I want to hear from YOU! Please feel free to send me an email with your thoughts, suggestions, and feedback regarding this book to talya@buddynsoul.com. I would love to hear what you think about this book and how it helped you with sticking to your pregnancy plan. Your feedback is extremely valuable and will allow us to help more individuals, like yourself, to obtain the necessary tools and support needed to change their lives for good.

What do you hope to gain from the Sticking to your Pregnancy Plan course?

You've decided to read this book. You're on board. What are some results you hope to come away with?

1. Becoming a more empowered patient throughout the pregnancy (yes, I'm a patient).
2. Doing a better job at sticking to my OB/GYN's diet, health, and medication requirements.
3. Feeling more in control of my body and how I take care of it.
4. A sense of excitement about my upcoming baby.
5. An increased sense of purpose and responsibility: knowing that what I do directly impacts my baby.

List some of your own ideas:

6. ____

7. ____

8. ____

Even as an expectant mama, you've got a baby to look after!

So much focus gets placed on mom-to-be and her belly, on the nursery and the name, that we sometimes forget about the star of the show: the very real baby growing in there.

Becoming pregnant is an adventure of transitions, as you experience multiple changes in your body, your lifestyle, and your relationships. All these changes are a reminder that your role has changed. That role, which began pre-conception and continues up until birth and beyond, is to nurture your baby as she grows within you.

But it's not always easy to remember that role, as we struggle with our own adjustments during pregnancy. **When you're trying to down a prenatal vitamin without throwing up, it's natural to be tempted to skip it – unless you can focus on what these vitamins mean to your baby.**

What you can do is remind yourself that the baby is a real person, with real needs that only you can meet. One way to make it real, to bring home the fact that your actions will affect your baby's health, is to visualize your baby as a real person.

Research shows that women who believe that they have an influence on the outcome of their pregnancy are more likely to make positive lifestyle changes and adhere to medical routines during pregnancy. When you visualize your beautiful baby after birth, let that image remind you what this is all about; why you are making such an effort to maintain your doctor's guidelines, restrictions and recommendations. You can influence the positive outcome of your pregnancy.

In the 'Exercise' component coming up, we will take the time to picture your baby after his or her birth. Try to make it real – to actually *see* your baby. Let that image serve as a positive reminder of how your current choices affect the development of that beautiful baby.

EXERCISE

Step 1: Close your eyes for a few moments and **imagine your baby** after his or her birth. Try to visualize a face, features, skin and hair color. Imagine you are touching his or her skin. Feel how soft it is. In your mind's eye, count your baby's fingers and toes and notice how perfectly formed he or she is. Use all your senses to really 'see' your baby.

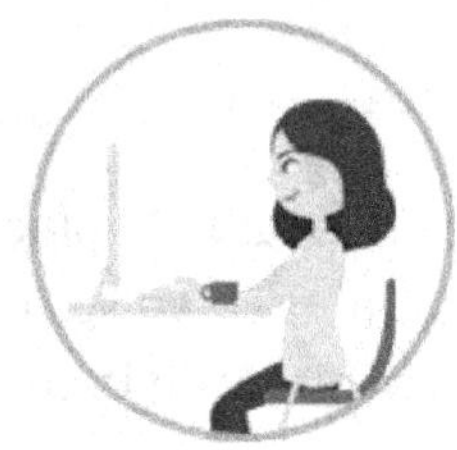

Step 2: Use your journal to write down a list of behaviors that are important to implement or avoid in order to **help your baby grow into that beautiful infant**. For example, you might put 'take my prenatal vitamins,' 'eat nutritious meals,' or 'drink no more than one coffee a day.'

TIPS

Tip 1: Some women find visualizing their baby very natural, while others have a hard time connecting their swollen belly with a newborn. Do your best. The main thing is to highlight to yourself that you are growing a real, beautiful baby inside you!

Tip 2: Don't know what to put on your list? Ask your OB/GYN what he/she recommends for a healthy pregnancy.

Visualization tips for the abstract thinking mama-to-be

Visualization is a great tool for all types of thinkers. For the abstract thinkers who naturally feel at ease with colors, shapes, and imaginative forms, here are some tips to enable you to soar with your visualizations and really bond with your upcoming baby.

1. Use your penchant for creative thinking to take your baby where no baby's gone before. Take her on wild adventures through space and time. Shrink down to her size and visit her in utero. The options are truly endless!
2. Ground your visualization with your breath. Start and end each visualization session by focusing on your breathing, which will in turn regulate your heartbeat.
3. Draw or write about your visualizations after the fact. You'll love reading them over with your child in a few years' time!

Do you have any tips?

4. ____

5. ____

6. ____

Visualization tips for the concrete mama-to-be

Visualization is a great tool, but some of us have a harder time getting into it than others. For the concrete thinkers among us who tend to do better with facts and figures, here are some tips to enable you to use visualization to help you bond with your baby.

1. Envision things about your baby that you know are there. You can use images you've seen online or from your ultrasound to help you.
2. Set a specific time for daily visualization. Knowing it's a legit part of your schedule will make it feel like a worthwhile pursuit.
3. Watch a sample video online to help you get a better idea of what visualization is all about. It will help you skip the self-judgment.
4. Think of it as a game. The less seriously you take yourself, the easier it'll be to get into the right headspace.

Do you have any tips?

5. ____

6. ____

7. ____

Visualizing my unborn baby is downright spooky, not helpful

I know visualizing the future is meant to be helpful. Yet when it comes to thinking about my unborn child I get the chills. It's one thing to see an ultrasound and another thing entirely to color in my child, so to speak.

For:

1. All I can think about are those cabbage patch doll heads and I get the shivers.
2. What's the point in envisioning something that I know will never actually be accurate? And then I'll be disappointed when my child is born without those delicious dimples I've imagined.
3. Haven't you ever heard of the 'evil eye?' This technique would definitely evoke it. And I would have brought it upon myself!

Add your own!

4. ____

Against:

1. My fetus is a part of me and is as real as I am. What's spooky about that?
2. I believe that thinking about and even visualizing my baby is part of the natural process of becoming a mother.
3. I think it would be spookier to *not* acknowledge my baby's presence

Add your own!

4. ____

Visualizing my baby helped me in a surprising way

Visualization simulates reality and can have surprising real-life results. What improvement did you experience in your pregnancy after visualizing your baby? Take a moment to reflect on your thoughts in your journal.

Direct message us YOUR story @Buddy_N_Soul on Instagram and be anonymously featured for a chance to **win a Buddy&Soul three month free membership.**

I'm glad that you've decided to learn more about sticking to your pregnancy plan with this book. Each section of this book consists of a warm-up talk, followed by a hands-on component where you'll learn a new skill or idea and have a chance to start putting it into action.

Watch 'The Battle Between Your Present and Future Self' presented by Daniel Goldstein on YouTube.

In this first TED Talk recommendation Daniel Goldstein explains how our behavior is affected by our awareness of and ability to imagine our future. If we can successfully imagine the future, that's a key tool in having the self-control we desire in the present.

He shares with us virtual reality software he developed to help make the future seem more real in key areas of life such as finances and health. As you watch the clip, consider whether you can visualize the effects of your behavior on your baby's health.

We think you'll find that the more you put into the course, the more you'll get out of it. So, take full advantage of all the resources and exercises and find your place in a community of people facing similar challenges.

9 Wishes I have for this pregnancy

When you're pregnant, there is so much to worry about, but so much to dream and fantasize about too. Focusing on your hopes and wishes can keep you sane, balanced, and positive during this potentially turbulent time. And the amazing thing about wishes is that they really can come true! Here are a few things every expectant mama wishes for.

1. **A healthy baby.** Just knowing I have that to look forward to carries me through all the pregnancy pains.
2. **A healthy mommy.** I want to come out healthy and strong at the end of this. I know that choices I make during pregnancy are critical in maintaining my postnatal health too.
3. **A strong relationship with my partner.** I hope we can thrive, and not only survive, through the strains of pregnancy.
   (Plus: Check out our Relationship Saver During Pregnancy course)
4. **An uneventful pregnancy.** Don't get me wrong, I love drama, but pregnancy is no time for added excitement. I'm hoping to fly under the radar and stick to boring old routine with this one.
5. **A body I feel good in.** Pregnancy is disorienting to say the least. I hardly recognize myself in the mirror from the shoulders down. Nonetheless, I hope I can go through this pregnancy feeling good about my body and myself.
6. **A smooth birth.** I don't care if it's early, late, induced, Caesarean, drug-filled or drug-free. The details are peripheral. Just let it lead to a healthy mom and a healthy baby!

Do you have any other wishes for your pregnancy?

7. ____

8. ____

9. ____

STRATEGY 2: Engage the power of your thoughts

In their book *Motivational Interviewing*, renowned researchers William Richard Miller and Stephen Rollnick explain that if you believe in your ability to make a change, you are much more likely to succeed.

What does this have to do with your pregnancy?

Well, you may believe that your doctor's recommendations are good for you and for your baby, but if your following thought is 'there's no way I'll be able to keep it up,' you likely won't stick to them all that closely.

Your thoughts influence your feelings, which influence your actions. If you think global warming is a sham, you probably won't conserve energy or recycle. Similarly, having a can-do attitude during pregnancy will improve your adherence, and that's a proven stat.

You'll need to buckle up, harness your positive thoughts, and believe in yourself. Believe that, yes, you can take your vitamins no matter how dizzy or nauseous you are. Yes, you can skip the spicy tuna maki no matter how mouthwatering it looks. And yes, you can limit your caffeine intake during pregnancy no matter how much you love your magic beans.

No one's saying it's gonna be easy, but believing is the first step toward achieving.

And here we're met with a bit of a philosophical conundrum: Can you change your thoughts about yourself? Either you have confidence in your ability to succeed, or you don't, right? Can anything be done to genuinely boost your confidence in your ability to do this and stick with it?

According to best-selling author and success expert Brian Tracy in *The Power of Self-Confidence,* the answer is a resounding yes! In his words, "Anything that you think about long enough and hard enough eventually becomes a part of your mental processes, exerting its influence and power on your attitude and your behavior" (p. 3).

You have the power to change your thoughts, boost your self-efficacy, and successfully adhere to your prenatal health plan.

With this in mind, let's pump up our can-do muscles by creating a positive mantra.

A mantra is a statement that you repeat to yourself because you want it to seep into your subconscious. It's usually stated in the present tense even if it's not 100% true yet and it affirms your belief of what you should be. For instance, 'I have iron-woman self-control and I do what is best for my baby and for me' or 'I get enough sleep each night and have eliminated my need for caffeine.'

When you develop your mantra, give yourself the benefit of the doubt. Work with the part of yourself that genuine believes in your ability follow your doctor's recommended health plan to a tee.

Creating a mantra that reflects your deep values is what makes it so powerful.

Find or create an empowering mantra about adhering to your prenatal lifestyle and/or health plan. It can be something like 'I nourish my baby with vitamins every day' or 'I am exercising moderately for 30 minutes most days of the week' or 'I abstain from alcohol because I love my baby.' Write your mantra in your journal.

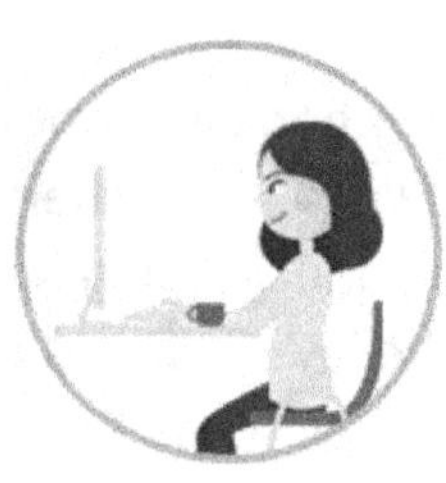

TIPS

Tip 1: Remember, you don't have to be doing it yet for it to be part of your mantra. Your mantra is what you are striving for!

Tip 2: Repeat your mantra at fixed times and situations, like while brushing your teeth. See our Habit Workshop course for more on introducing new habits into your daily routine.

Tip 3: Revisit your journal any time to modify, revise, or add to your mantra.

Positive mantras won't help my adherence

There are all these great techniques out there that help with adherence. But mantras? Seriously? That won't have any bearing on how well I adhere to my doctor's prenatal requirements.

For:

1. I'm not into things like mantras and chakras and kombucha and what not.
2. Positive, you say? Well, I'm more of a realistic type. And I don't think a mantra about how utterly unmotivated I'm feeling is quite what I'm supposed to be after here.
3. Nothing can help my stick to my pregnancy plan. I'm totally doomed!

Add your own idea!

4. ____

Against:

1. What do I have to lose? Even if I think it sounds hokey, it takes only a few seconds. No harm in trying.
2. A mantra can be both realistic and positive. It can reflect my struggles, but also my higher aspirations. There is no contradiction there.
3. Positive mantras are a great idea. They have helped me in other areas. Maybe they could help here too.

Add your own idea!

4. ____

Things I gained by sticking to my prenatal regimen

Sometimes, challenging yourself to stick to something that you know will help you has far-reaching results in other areas of your life. In addition to the obvious medical benefits of adherence, what have you gained from following your prenatal regimen to a tee?

1. **Owning it.** I learned to put on my big badge and swallow my bitter pill.
2. **Responsible self-bribery.** I can maturely offer myself some rewards without falling off the wagon.
3. **A sense of accomplishment.** It feels good to do the right thing, especially when it doesn't come naturally.
4. **Perspective.** I am not the only one being impacted my decisions. I'm part of something much larger than myself.
5. **Empowerment.** When I do what's right even though it's not fun or easy, I feel stronger somehow. Like I can face whatever comes my way. Yes, I am woman. Hear me roar!

What can you gain from sticking to your prenatal regimen?

6. ____

7. ____

8. ____

My pregnancy adherence mantra that really made a difference

The messages we say to ourselves have a powerful influence on our feelings and behaviors. What mantra helps you make healthy decisions during your pregnancy? Write more about it in your journal.

Direct message us YOUR mantra @Buddy_N_Soul on Instagram and be anonymously featured for a chance to **win a Buddy&Soul three month free membership.**

DRIVING THE MESSAGE HOME

Brian Tracy is Chairman and CEO of Brian Tracy International, a company specializing in the training and development of individuals and organizations. He is an entrepreneur, public speaker, best-selling author and success expert. When it comes to believing in yourself and your capabilities, he is an absolute pro.

Watch 'Change Your Life for the Better' presented by Brian Tracy on YouTube.

Listen to Tracy's take on the three main obstacles to self-confidence and his thoughts about how confidence, or lack thereof, will influence your thoughts and behaviors.

Spoiler alert: If your confidence is low, your ability to stick to your medical recommendations will probably be low too, whether or not you're pregnant.

So, give yourself a confidence boost and an adherence boost, and move towards better prenatal health for you and your baby.

How low self-confidence was impacting my prenatal health

Low self-confidence can hold you back from trying to achieve your dreams. If low self-confidence was getting in the way during your pregnancy, think about your experience and what you learned from it! Take five minutes to write in your journal about this lesson.

(Plus: Check out our Claim Your Self-Esteem course 🙂 for more.)

Direct message us YOUR story @Buddy_N_Soul on Instagram and be anonymously featured for a chance to **win a Buddy&Soul three month free membership.**

STRATEGY 3: Up your knowledge base

If you're like most pregnant women, you're already worrying about your baby. And how could you not? The mire of information available these days could cause even your Himalayan meditation instructor to panic.

And yet, when it comes to health, diet, and medications during pregnancy, it's crucial to get a handle on the facts rather than making rash or uninformed decisions.

Research from the Departments of Pediatrics and Medicine at the Children's Hospital in London, Ontario highlights just how important accurate prenatal health information is.

Their study found that many pregnant women skip taking prescribed meds because they *erroneously* believe the meds will harm their baby. Lacking evidence-based information from their healthcare providers, they fill in the gaps based on misconceptions, which can have detrimental effects to say the least.

So, **before you skip a pill, a med, a vaccination, or ignore a dietary requirement because you're certain it's the right thing to do, do your research.**

And that means from reliable sources. Ahem.

Your doctor, midwife, or doula should be a great starting point. But, Alice Domar and Sheila Oakes, authors of *Finding Calm for the Expectant Mom* (2016), caution women about information found online, as many sites are not monitored for accuracy (p. 49).

If you're unsure about something you've been prescribed, the best thing to do is seek out information and get back to your doctor or midwife with questions.

Some things to consider are:

- Why you've been prescribed a particular medication, supplement, or vitamin
- What the alternatives are
- What the research says about this treatment's safety for pregnant women
- How easy is it to take, how often you have to take it, and what to do if you slip up, miss a dose, etc.
- What the possible side effects are and when to call a medical professional
- When you can you expect to see results from this treatment
- What happens if you don't follow the plan as prescribed
- Anything else you might want to know

Reminder: Don't be shy when it's your health that's under discussion. And you are not hurting anyone's feelings by asking questions. This is your body and your baby; you are entitled to all the information in the world.

Strengthen your ability to stick to your pregnancy plan by upping your knowledge-base. The more you know, the more power and confidence you will have in this journey, and the greater the chances will be that you'll successfully adhere to your doctor's pregnancy guidelines.

EXERCISE

Step 1: **Rate your knowledge of your pregnancy requirements.** How true is each
of these statements for you? Take a few minutes to reflect in your journal.

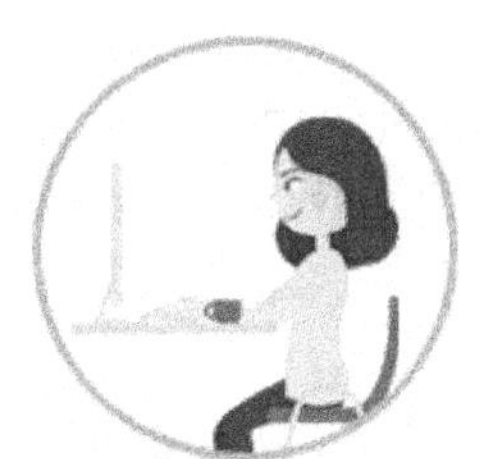

1. I know all about the vitamins and supplements I should be taking.
2. I know all about the dietary changes I need to make.
3. I know all about the prescription medications or hormones I need to take.
4. I know all about the over-the-counter products I need to avoid.
5. I know all about the lifestyle tweaks that are required for my pregnancy.

Step 2: If you strongly agreed with all five statements – good for you! You may pass Go and
proceed to the next session.

If you disagreed or strongly disagreed with any of the statements, use your journal to
identify what more you'd need to find out to bring your knowledge base up. **Prepare a list of
questions to take with you to your next prenatal visit.**

TIPS

Tip 1: Schedule some time into your calendar to research and fill in the information gaps. It
doesn't have to be a huge block of time. Just get it done. Commit to it and follow through.

Tip 2: Some websites and apps gather patient feedback about medication. Check out our
app recommendations to see what's being said about any meds you're taking.

Tip 3: You can use your journal to log new info you come across as you maneuver your way
through the book.

8 Ways knowledge can help you stick to your pregnancy plan

When you understand the purpose of your pregnancy routine, you'll have the courage to stick with it. Here's why…

1. If you don't know why you're keeping up a prenatal routine, it's much harder to stay motivated. You've got to understand the benefits of what you are doing.
2. You've heard the saying "knowledge is power." When you know why you're doing something, you are aware of how your actions affect your future.
3. When I learned about what could happen to my baby if I didn't take my folic acid (i.e. spina bifida, a malformation of his spine), I took my pill every day, religiously.
4. It's crucial to learn about mother and fetal health during pregnancy. What you do now can affect your baby for a very long time.
5. Researching your doctor's recommendations provides you with an opportunity to learn about alternative options, and then ask about them. Many doctors will be open to discussing different good options with you during your pregnancy.

How can knowledge help you?

6. ____

7. ____

8. ____

Does knowledge increase adherence to medical treatment?

Education is the usual go-to for changing behavior. And yet we still find no shortage of smokers, drunk drivers, or people engaging in unsafe sex who know full well what the ramifications of their choices may be. So, what's to say that if I knew better about my pregnancy plan I would be any better at sticking to it?

For:

1. Of course it does. The more I know, the more my knowledge influences my behavior.
2. I'm convinced that if someone would take the time to explain the medical basis that underlies my prenatal plan, my adherence would be forever improved.
3. Humans can think things through. Our neocortex sets us apart from animals. Let's use it!

Add your own idea:

4. ____

Against:

1. Knowledge is important, yes. But at the end of the day, I prefer to go with my gut instinct.
2. I know I should be sticking to my pregnancy plan, and I don't. More knowledge would simply lead to more contradictory behavior. I'm not proud of it, but c'est la vie.
3. What about all the emotional richness we all possess? I, for one, am more motivated by the emotional bond with my baby than by facts and figures. There is more to sticking to my plan than knowledge.

Add your own idea:

4. ____

The piece of info that turned my prenatal health around

It might seem insignificant to someone else, but to you, it made all the difference. Think about that tip, insight, or fact that had a positive impact on your prenatal health. Write more about it in your journal.

Direct message us YOUR insights @Buddy_N_Soul on Instagram and be anonymously featured for a chance to **win a Buddy&Soul three month free membership.**

DRIVING THE MESSAGE HOME

There's a lot of discussion today about patient-centered medicine versus doctor-centered medicine. If the expertise flowing from doctors to patients, should the doctors be the ones making all the decisions? How much involvement should patients have?

Pregnancy is *not* a disease but it *is* a condition that requires medical attention.

Watch 'Who is the Real Medical Expert?' presented by Roni Zeiger on tedmed.com

In a talk from Roni Zeiger, M.D., he gives several examples of how patients, who have become experts in the science of their conditions, have banded together to make rather impressive advances.

Zeiger left his position as the former Chief Health Strategist at Google and, together with Gilles Frydman, founded 'Smart Patients' in order to amplify the knowledge created by networks of engaged patients.

As you watch, think about how all of this relates to pregnancy, and to *your* pregnancy in particular. How informed are you about the medical side of things? And how involved are you in decisions regarding mama and baby's health?

There's lots to think about. And here we go!

Ways to get the most out of your prenatal visits

You're going to a plethora of prenatal appointments *anyway* – you might as well get the most out of them! Here are a few ideas for starters.

1. If you're feeling timid, think of the least shy person you know and pretend to be them. Tell yourself "I'm doing this for my baby."
2. Write out your list of questions *in advance*. A prepared mama-to-be leads to a productive prenatal appointment.
3. Take your partner or someone you trust along with you for the weightier appointments, like the fetal scan or any diagnostic tests. You might need some extra moral support.
4. Inquire about the best way to reach your OB/GYN or midwife between appointments. Questions will invariably arise along the way and you'll want to make sure you have an address to turn to for reliable answers.
5. Take notes! Don't rely on your memory (especially not these days…).
6. Listen to your instincts. If you're unhappy with the care you're receiving or if something about it feels off, don't rush to silence that voice. No patient-physician relationship is perfect, but you should absolutely feel comfortable with your care.

Any other suggestions?

7. ____

8. ____

9. ____

Pregnancy hasn't been exactly what you expected, has it? (No pun intended.)

Yes, being pregnant is wonderful. And yet, you might find yourself sulking occasionally as you long for elements of your carefree, non-pregnant life.

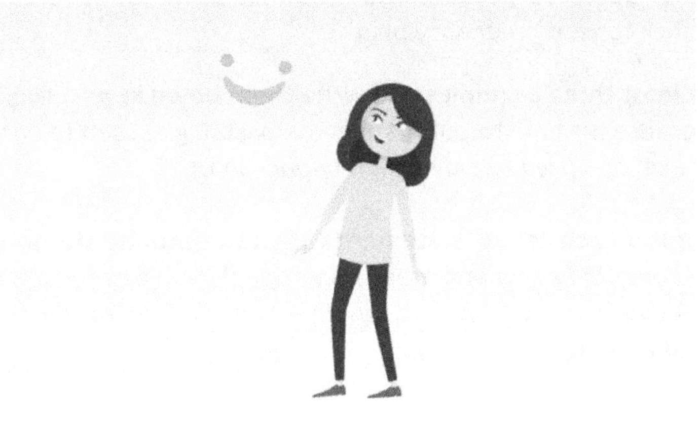

You used to drink socially, and now it's a no-no. You love to go skiing, and this winter it's out. The doctor is telling you to limit your weight gain, and you can't seem to stomach anything but donuts. It just doesn't seem fair that so much of your lifestyle has to change, even though you want to do what's best for baby.

So, what do you do?

Well, first, **it's time to actively let go of your expectations of what pregnancy should or shouldn't look like**.

For instance, you always knew pregnancy meant no alcohol, but the no donuts thing really threw you off! Recognizing that can help you recalibrate.

Next, you need to tap into a new mindset – one that celebrates what a difference you are making to your baby's health. Pinpoint any unrealistic expectations or behaviors you need to let go of and imagine them fading away, flowing downriver.

Remind yourself that this is a new curve in the journey and you are adapting to a new role. Actually, adjusting your mindset is good preparation for parenthood, which will certainly bring new changes to your life.

Once you've changed your mindset by letting go, it can be helpful to replace the old with something new. Put some thought into what energizes and invigorates you in this stage (pregnancy-compatible of course!).

If you're not drinking anymore, what can you do or have that feels like an indulgence? Although you might not be able to ski, can you find another activity that pumps up your energy, like a dance class?

Once you let go of the expectations and tap into a more positive mindset, you might be surprised to find strengths and interests you never knew you had.

EXERCISE

Step 1: What lifestyle expectations are you holding on to that are making it harder to stick to your pregnancy plan?

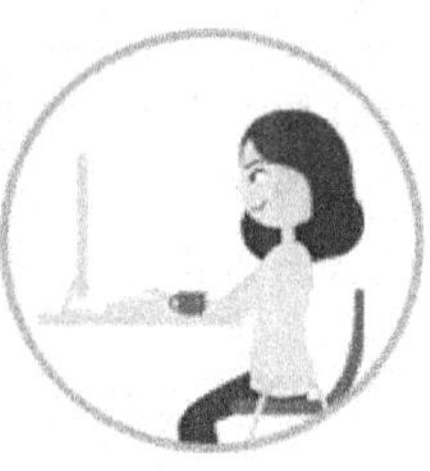

Identify at least three examples and write them down in past tense in your journal, because it's time to put them in the past. E.g. *'I used to eat or drink what I felt like'* or *'I used to play a high-impact sport.'*

Step 2: **Counter each 'let go' statement with a turnaround statement** – a statement suggesting something new and pregnancy-friendly you can do to replace what you're letting go of. E.g. *'I have cool non-alcoholic drinks when I go out,'* or *'I'm buying tickets to watch the sports I used to play.'*

TIPS

Tip 1: Remind yourself that most pregnancy-related lifestyle tweaks are temporary, and you'll probably be able to resume them later on.

Tip 2: Check out our _Declutter Your Mind course_ for more on letting go of unhelpful expectations.

7 Reasons I hate taking my prenatal vitamins!

The doctor has prescribed them and you know you should take them but you really wish you didn't have to! Here are some of the reasons:

1. It's just one more thing to remember during this pregnancy when I'm already having a hard enough time doing everything.
2. It makes me feel as if my pregnancy is a medical condition instead of something amazing and wonderful.
3. They make me so nauseous!
4. They're always coming out with new studies. What happens if it turns out they discover that I've been taking too much stuff? Or even worse, something harmful.

Add your own:

5. ____

6. ____

7. ____

Hardest things to let go of when you're pregnant

There are so many life changes you need to make when you're pregnant in order to optimize your and your baby's health. The fact that it's only temporary doesn't help when all you want is a sunny side up egg with a runny yolk. What are some of the hardest changes you've had to make?

1. My favorite foods, like hot dogs and sushi.
2. High-risk sports like snowboarding, scuba diving, or mountain biking.
3. Drinking.
4. Smoking.
5. Sleeping on my back.

What are going to be your hardest changes?

6. ____

7. ____

8. ____

What happened when I dropped my pregnancy expectations

You thought…you planned…you expected… But all that was before you were expecting. Now that you're actually pregnant, you've had to drop a variety of unrealistic expectations. Reflect in your journal on what that was like, and how you have learned to go with the flow in pregnancy.

Direct message us YOUR story @Buddy_N_Soul on Instagram and be anonymously featured for a chance to **win a Buddy&Soul three month free membership.**

Watch 'Letting go of Expectations' presented by Heather Marshall at TEDxGreenville on YouTube.

In the next suggested TED talk, writer and teacher Heather Marshall walks us through the lessons she learned about expectations on her search for her biological parents.

Our expectations shape our inner world. They tell us how things should be. The problem is that they often don't match with reality, and then we get stuck.

Marshall discusses the importance of letting go in relationships, but her message holds true in other areas of life as well.

As you watch this, think about what pregnancy-related expectations you're holding to and whether you can let them go.

8 Expectations I had going into pregnancy

There's a big difference between aspirations and expectations. Aspirations are hopeful and motivational, but expectations? Not so much. The negative ones prime us for anxiety and the positive ones set us up for disappointment. What are some of your pesky expectations – negative or positive – that may be impacting your satisfaction levels during your pregnancy?

1. I'm going to look like Demi Moore on the cover of Vanity Fair. Or better!
2. Nausea is for the weak. I'm going to feel like the Energizer Bunny my entire pregnancy.
3. I'm going to perfectly adhere to every part of my pregnancy plan, including a strict exercise, diet, and vitamin regimen. No midwife has ever seen an expectant mom quite like me.
4. Pregnancy is all about worrying. I expect myself to be a nervous wreck from the moment I discover I'm expecting until well after the birth. Or, after the baby stage. Or at least after the toddler years. Or, scrap that, after my kid learns to drive… Hm…
5. I expect my prenatal decisions to be taken care of for me. I won't have to take ownership or get informed about pregnancy requirements – the ball is in my OB/GYN's court. After all, she's the expert, is she not?

What expectations did you have?

6. ____

7. ____

8. ____

STRATEGY 5: Identify your prenatal adherence hurdles

When your OB/GYN prescribes a medication or treatment plan, she usually focuses on the drug's medical benefits: iron to help your body make extra blood for you and your baby, folic acid to prevent birth defects, and foods with a low GI to keep your blood sugars down.

Of course, the medical rationale is of primary importance, since you're not going to take medication that doesn't benefit you and your baby. And yet, often this isn't enough to get you to actually stick to the plan.

There are other, less critical factors that influence your motivation and ability to adhere.

Let's figure this out. **Why wouldn't a pregnant woman be 100% adherent to doctor's orders concerning her pregnancy?** She does want what's best for her and her baby, doesn't she?

Well, it's not that simple. And a study from the Tuck Business School at Dartmouth College demonstrates just how complex it can get. They found that each of the following practical factors can contribute to patient adherence, or lack thereof:

- How immediately you can see the results of your meds
- How easy the medication is to take
- How much you have to pay out-of-pocket
- The existence and intensity of side effects – both in terms of their frequency and severity

Indeed, pregnant women participating in a study in Tanzania were found to be a third less likely to take their pills if they experienced side effects.

Any of this sound familiar?

Social and emotional factors can impact your adherence as well. For instance:

- Your level of control in the decision-making process
- Peer pressure to fit in with your pre-pregnancy crowd
- Cultural factors, like a societal belief that pregnant women "should not take any medication"
- How well the treatment or lifestyle change fits in with your lifestyle and existing habits

Whether technical or emotional, you want to identify what factors are making it harder for you to follow *your* prenatal guidelines so you can nip them in the bud.

Let's take some time now to explore what, if anything, is hindering your ability to stick to your pregnancy plan. And then let's start working on solutions.

EXERCISE

Step 1: **Decide what interferes with your ability to optimally stick to your pregnancy plan?**

1. I don't believe my prenatal regimen is necessary or helpful.
2. There are bothersome side effects.
3. Sticking to my prenatal treatment plan is expensive.
4. The meds I need are challenging to take (injections, IVs, "horse pills").
5. I resist change in general.
6. I often slip up or forget.
7. My prenatal regimen interferes with my lifestyle.
8. I feel societal pressure to be "au naturel" during pregnancy.
9. I don't feel I was part of the medical decision-making process.
10. I don't want to feel like I'm ill. After all, pregnancy is a sign of wellness!

Step 2: Consider the answers you rated the highest. Now, **brainstorm a list of ways to circumvent or solve the issues.**

For example, maybe you need to take iron, but the side effects are unpleasant. Work-arounds could be to crowdsource and find out how other people solved the problem, or to investigate different sources of iron you could take.

List your work-around ideas in your journal.

TIPS

Tip 1: Social and cultural pressures can be very subtle. Remember that there are as many ways to do a healthy pregnancy as there are pregnant women. Don't get stuck on what society tells you is *the* way.

Tip 2: Sometimes, doing what we know is right simply comes down to having adequate willpower. Check out our Willpower 101 course for more on building that muscle!

Emotional hurdles of sticking to your pregnancy plan

Pregnancy is a time of your life when your hormones are raging and you're full of emotions. The following emotions can really act as stumbling blocks when it comes to sticking to your pregnancy plan.

1. **Shame.** There must be something wrong with me that I need to take 'stick to a plan' during this pregnancy. I've heard of plenty of people who were never told to take anything. Why can others just have it all natural and easy?
1. **Embarrassment.** What will my friends think when they see me popping pills, even if they are only prenatal vitamins and folic acid? I'm not ready to tell everyone I'm pregnant!
2. **Anger.** I'm a grown up and a free spirit. Why do I need to follow a plan? I'm mad at my doctor. I'm mad at myself. I'm mad at the world. I'm too mad to talk right now. And definitely too mad to stick to a plan.
3. **Guilt.** I know I should be sticking to my pregnancy plan and I'm not. If something happens to me or my baby it's going to be my fault.
4. Sadness. I can't help but mourn the loss of my freedom. I can no longer do as I please because someone else is depending on me at every moment.
5. **Denial.** I am sticking to my plan...more or less. It's okay if I cut corners every now and again.

Can you think of any other hurdles?

6. ____

7. ____

8. ____

What's the hardest part of sticking to your prenatal requirements?

Sticking to your doctor's orders is challenging at the best of times, and even tougher when you're pregnant. Here are some of the most common reasons patients generally find it tough to adhere. How much does each relate to your challenges in sticking to your prenatal health plan?

1. I don't feel immediate results when I do stick to the plan.
2. Adhering requires considerable effort.
3. It's expensive.
4. There are unpleasant side effects.
5. I have little or no sense of ownership in the decision-making process.
6. Peer pressure to fit in with my pre-pregnancy crowd and way of life.
7. Cultural factors, like a societal belief that pregnant women "should not take any medication."
8. The required treatment or lifestyle change clashes with my lifestyle and existing habits.

What do you think is the hardest part of sticking to your prenatal requirements?

9. ____

10. ____

11. ____

With the best of intentions, you might still battle adherence during pregnancy, and for any of a million reasons. Once you are aware of what's going on, it's possible to do something about it. What was getting in your way of adherence?

This section of the book is going to have you questioning what holds you back from optimally sticking to your pregnancy plan. Or, in other words, why do so many of us find it so challenging to follow our doctor's prescribed pregnancy routine?

In the TED talk presented by psychologist Barry Schwartz he talks about the paradox of choice and how the more choices we have, the more unhappy we become.

Watch 'The Paradox of Choice' presented by Barry Schwartz on www.ted.com.

As you're watching think about how your own adherence would look if you knew there was just one option available to you.

10 Surprising ideas about the paradox of choice

In his TED Talk *The Paradox of Choice,* psychologist Barry Schwartz makes some pretty radical claims. Here are some ideas – from the talk and elsewhere – that might sound counter-intuitive but are proven to throw things like choice and decision out the window. These all have implications for how well you stick to your pregnancy plan!

1. More choice does not equal more freedom. In fact, it equals paralysis.
2. Patient autonomy can be negative when you shift responsibility from the doctor who is informed and knowledgeable to the patient who is sick, or uncomfortably pregnant, and not necessarily in the best shape to make decisions.
3. People can accomplish less in their lives than in the past because they are preoccupied with making important choices.
4. Almost everything in life is a choice nowadays. That's a whole lot of choice!
5. Too much choice almost inevitably ends in being unhappy with the choice that was made. Think about it, there's always another option, or another option, or another option to have doubts about.
6. Too much choice means constantly living with a fear of missing out.
7. With every choice, our expectations get higher and higher.

What else did you learn?

8. ____

9. ____

10. ____

9 Motivators to help you stick to your pregnancy plan

Following your doctor's orders is tough at the best of times – throw in some wacky hormones and morning sickness and anyone will agree you have a good excuse to slip up here and there. You know it's important to keep your game tight, but sometimes it's hard to remember why. Allow us jog your memory.

1. The primary motivator for many is the future health of their yet unborn baby – the risk-reduction associated with proper prenatal care, etc.
2. Many women are motivated by the direct benefits they see to their health, like fewer leg cramps when they take the proper mineral supplements, or the ability to sustain a pregnancy when they take their prescribed hormones.
3. Knowing that you've followed all the rules and done things "right" takes the guilt and pressure off – you've done all that's in your hands and that's all you can do.
4. It gives you at least a semblance of control within all the unpredictability of pregnancy.
5. There's that rewarding feeling of doing something selfless for the sake of your child (amplified, as your baby has yet to be born).
6. Of course, life offers no guarantees, but if the science overwhelmingly supports your doctor's instructions, it's probably a safe place to bet your chips.

Add your own motivators:

7. ____

8. ____

9. ____

STRATEGY 6: Get some support

If you're like most people, you'll probably find that the Beatles were onto something when they claimed you'd get by with a little help from your friends.

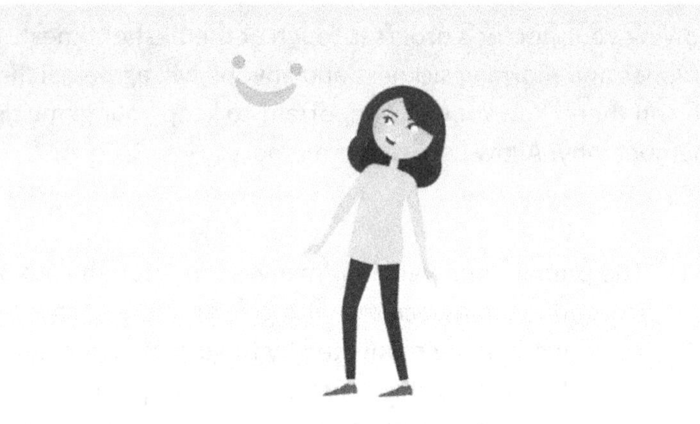

That's because it's universally true that emotional support can ease a tough time. And pregnancy is no exception.

Even if your pregnancy has been as smooth as that aged Tennessee whiskey your doctor keeps categorically prohibiting (for good reason, but still…), it's a time of transition – a new turn on the journey of your life.

Support not only feels good but actually has positive physiological effects, energizing and strengthening your body. A study conducted by researchers at Vanderbilt's Peabody Research Institute concluded that group prenatal care had "statistically and clinically significant beneficial effects."

According to lead author of the study, Emily E. Tanner-Smith, "putting women in supportive environments leads to increased happiness and improved outcomes." What this means practically is that interacting with a supportive community during your pregnancy can be good for you and your baby.

Even more important than community support is individual social support. In another study, researchers from Brazil and England found that pregnant women who had higher levels of individual support were more likely to stop smoking and eat healthier.

So here's the bottom line: **Maintaining your connections with supportive people will help you stick to your prenatal health plan.**

There's no one right way to go about it; emotional support means different things for different people. It can come from community, marriage or partnership, friends, pets, religion, a therapist or coach, to name a few.

In the 'Exercise' component that follows, we'll look at what emotional support means for you and do a little brainstorming to increase the level of emotional support that you're receiving during your pregnancy.

EXERCISE

Step 1: **Gain clarity on what emotional support means for you**. Answer the following questions in your journal:

- What makes you feel validated and supported during pregnancy?
- What type of support do you have but wish you had a bit more of?
- What type of support are you lacking?

Step 2: Now that you've articulated what kinds of support you have and lack, **brainstorm a list of ideas to increase your level of emotional support.** How can you get more of what you need?

For example, if you feel supported when you talk to other pregnant women, you might like to sign up for a group with other expectant mamas. Or, if talking to your sister makes you feel validated, maybe you can schedule a regular phone date.

TIPS

Tip 1: For some people, the kind of emotional support they enjoyed pre-pregnancy still works. Other women might be looking for something a little different during pregnancy.

Tip 2: If you like the idea of turning to your partner for support, you'll love our Relationship Saver During Pregnancy course!

8 Suggestions to help you join online pregnancy support groups

Perhaps joining an online support group sounds like a fine plan, but with so many options out there, it can be hard to know where to begin! These suggestions should help you get a good start.

1. Start here! Check out BuddynSoul.com and our Pregnancy & Birth community for starters. This way you can get support and practice the courses together.
2. Get specific about your needs. Figuring out what kind of support would best suit you is step one. For example, are you struggling with a particular aspect of pregnancy or the shabang? Do you want a forum where you can be anonymous, or post as yourself? Ask yourself some questions before you begin your search.
3. Court your suitors. Spend some time poking around the Internet before committing to any one support group or forum. Because any meaningful commitment is preceded by a period of courtship.
4. Introduce yourself. Regardless of what you've determined as your online identity, make sure to say a little about yourself and what you're looking for when you join. This is a great way to break the ice.
5. Be helpful where you can. When people recognize you (i.e. your avatar) as someone who supports others, they'll be more inclined to "be there" for you too.

Add your own ideas:

6. ____

7. ____

8. ____

What traits do you look for in your pregnancy support people?

There are so many well-intending people out there. What sets apart those who can really help us stick to our pregnancy plan?

47

1. **Altruistic.** How much are they thinking about helping me vs. helping themselves?
2. **Caring.** How much do they care about me?
3. **Strong-willed.** How much do they challenge me to do better?
4. **Trust-worthy.** Have they earned my trust over time?
5. **Emotionally savvy.** Do they make room for my emotions? Can they handle me?

What other traits do you value?

6. ____

7. ____

8. ____

How support helped me improve my prenatal health

We all need good people around us, especially during pregnancy when life is rapidly changing and emotions are sky-high. How did your support system bolster you and your health during your pregnancy? Take five minutes to write about it in your journal.

Direct message us YOUR story @Buddy_N_Soul on Instagram and be anonymously featured for a chance to **win a Buddy&Soul three month free membership.**

Do you have a person in your life with whom you feel close enough to share a personal problem? Someone you can turn to for support when the going gets really rough?

If your answer is yes, that's wonderful.

Astonishingly, though, for more and more people, the answer is a lonely no, as we discover at the beginning of Emma Seppälä's TEDx talk.

Watch 'The Power & Science of Social Connection' presented by Emma Seppälä on YouTube.

Seppälä shares with us the physical and emotional impacts of isolation versus healthy social connections. She explains the science behind how we can strengthen the relationships in our own lives.

As you watch, consider what kinds of social and emotional support you're receiving during your pregnancy and how you can build on that.

Because, especially when you're pregnant but even when you're not, a little emotional support goes a long way.

What helps you stick to your prenatal health plan?

Just like there are factors that deter you from sticking to your pregnancy plan, there are also factors that contribute to you sticking to your health plan. If you know what works for you, then keep on doing it. It can only help you when it comes to your overall adherence.

1. I feel better when I take my pills.
2. Support from my friends and loved ones.
3. I know it's important.
4. I am terrified of my doctor.
5. I'm so used to it by now. It's become a habit.
6. My strong willpower.

Is there anything else that helps you?

7. ____

8. ____

9. ____

STRATEGY 7: Rate your conscientiousness level

Whether or not you're pregnant, sticking to any kind of medical plan or health regimen is a challenge.

Finding one variable that would accurately predict your likelihood to succeed at adhering would be a game-changer. And whaddya know – psychologists Brent Roberts of the University of Illinois and Patrick Hill of Washington University have done just that.

According to their research, the key ingredient to predict adherence is a character trait that we all possess to some extent or other: conscientiousness, a.k.a. the tendency to stick with rules and regimens.

In their words, "conscientious individuals report higher levels of both doctor and medication adherence."

That means if you're one of those people who *will* follow instructions to a tee come Hell or high water, you'll probably find you're in the clear when it comes to sticking to your pregnancy plan too.

That's happy news for conscientious folks, but where exactly does that leave the rest of us? You know, those of us who are more prone to breaking rules, or shelving them for an evening, a day, or as long as it feels good? Are we automatically doomed to poor adherence if we don't possess this magical trait in heaping portions?

The answer is a resounding no!

You might have your work cut out for you, but rest assured it can be done.

While it's true that some lucky people are super conscientious by nature, the rest of us *can* work on ourselves to develop this skill.

For starters, remember that it's not an all-or-nothing scenario. Conscientiousness is a scale. Very few people, if any, have *zero* conscientiousness in them. That means that you likely already have something to work with, which is a big plus. You can build on isolated successes you've had and take it from there, step by step.

Next, keep in mind that your level of conscientiousness is a lever, not an excuse. Use it to help guide your adherence efforts and catapult you forward. That means that if you're naturally less conscientious, you'll work a little harder to maintain full adherence.

The lower your conscientiousness score, the more help you'll need (such as setting up a reminder system), and the more committed you'll have to decide to be.

In any case, **once you know how conscientious you are or aren't, you can start working with your natural tendencies and find effective ways to stick to your pregnancy plan.**

Use your score to choose the tips and tricks that will help you push your adherence higher.

The end goal is that you feel better and have better health outcomes, and that is worth it – for you and your baby.

EXERCISE

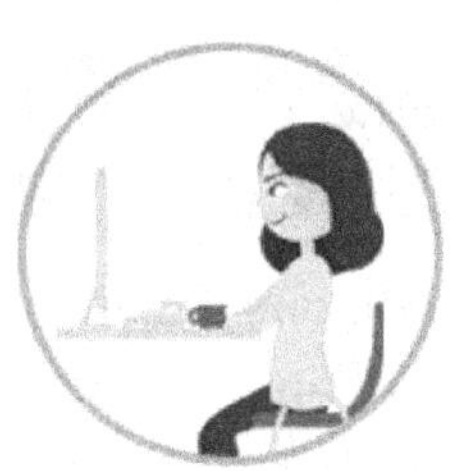

Step 1: Respond to the questionnaire below to find out your level of consciousness. Read each of the following statements and rate the level at which you agree on a scale of 1 to 4, with 1 being strongly disagree and 4 being strongly agree.

(Source: Based on Roberts, B. W., Walton, K. E., & Bogg, T. (2005). Conscientiousness and health across the life course. *Review of General Psychology,* 9(2), 156.)

1. I am easily talked into doing silly things
2. I support long-established rules and traditions
3. I rarely jump into something without first thinking about it
4. I do not intend to follow every little rule that others make up
5. I often rush into action without thinking about potential consequences
6. Even if I knew how to get around the rules without breaking them, I would not do it
7. I am careful what I say to others
8. When I was in school, I used to break rules quite regularly

Scorecard:

	What you ranked yourself:			
	1	2	3	4
Question #:	What it's worth: (for overall summary)			
1.	4	3	2	1
2.	1	2	3	4
3.	1	2	3	4
4.	4	3	2	1
5.	4	3	2	1
6.	1	2	3	4
7.	1	2	3	4
8.	4	3	2	1
TOTAL:				

Now that you've rated each statement, check the scorecard to see how many points you've got. Add up your points to come up with a total, and see where you fall on the Conscientiousness scale, below:

- High Conscientiousness is between 24 - 32
- Medium Conscientiousness is between 16 – 23
- Low Conscientiousness is between   8 - 15

Step 2: Is your score congruent with the way you see yourself? **What is your impression of how your level of conscientiousness helps or hinders your ability to stick to your prenatal health plan?** Write your answers in your journal.

Tip 1: If you're low on conscientiousness, check out our Willpower 101 course to help give you a self-control boost.

Tip 2: Don't be discouraged by a low score! It means that now you can better address the problem areas to maximize your adherence.

Should I even bother working on adherence to my pregnancy plan?

I wasn't born with the gift of a conscientious personality and following rules has never been my modus operandi. Is there even any point in my trying to up my game now? Seems kinda pointless.

For:

1. Adherence is a skill. All skills are learned. I got this.
2. Dude, it's my baby's health we're talking about. If this isn't worth making an effort for, I don't know what is.
3. It's all about willpower and self-control. If I believe in my pregnancy plan, I can follow it.
4. If my doctor prescribed a daily scoop of ice cream at 8pm every night, I bet my "old dog" would learn that "new trick" in record time! I'll just make believe I enjoy my pregnancy plan as much I love eating ice cream.
5. There's a sense of accomplishment in knowing *I made a change* – I used to forget all the time, but now sticking to my plan is like a second nature.

Add an additional benefit of working on adherence to your pregnancy plan:

6. ____

Against:

1. Adherence is something you're either born with or not. I wasn't born with it. The end.
2. I am who I am. When I push myself beyond my capabilities, it doesn't last. I'll get in maybe a month or two of good adherence at best, and then it's back to my old ways.
3. At a time like this, when I'm facing so make challenge and change, I need to go easy on myself. It's not that I think it's right or responsible, I just don't need to get into a shame spiral about it.
4. Thinking of change gives me the jitters. (Plus: Check out our Tackling Change course)

Add your own idea:

5. ____

Adherence struggles faced by not-so-conscientious mamas-to-be

When it comes to sticking to your pregnancy plan, we'd all love to fall into that super-conscientious category where following through is easy and automatic. However, we're not all that lucky, and when you're pregnant and tired, it only gets worse! Here are some common adherence struggles those moms-to-be with a less than perfect conscientious score face.

1. **Guilt.** When you're making decisions for one, it's one thing. But when you know your decisions impact your baby and you *still* can't get it together, well, that's a tough pill to swallow (so to speak).
2. **Disorientation.** If you generally like to be spontaneous and make decisions on the fly, it can be tremendously disorienting to transition to a new mode that involves planning ahead and being very organized. If you feel off-kilter or out of sorts with the new you, rest assured you are not alone.
   (Sometimes, we have to put aside our authenticity for a greater good. Check out our Cultivating Authenticity course for more).
3. **Stifling.** For those mamas-to-be who struggle with rule-following, adhering to a pregnancy plan can feel tremendously stifling. You know it's a worthy cause but you can't help but wonder where your freedom has gone…
4. **Anger.** Let's face it – adherence is friggin' hard, especially when it doesn't come naturally. It's okay to be angry at all the demands that pregnancy places upon you!

What are some struggles that you believe will become an obstacle?

5. ____

6. ____

7. ____

Know thyself – because awareness goes a long way towards change. How have you had an easier time sticking to your pregnancy plan after learning your conscientiousness score? Take some time to reflect in your journal.

When it comes to sticking to your medical or dietary regimens during pregnancy, certain personality traits can make it easier or harder.

As we'll explore in the activity that follows the next TED talk, one of the most predictive traits is conscientiousness. By looking at a person's level of conscientiousness, along with their other major traits, you can gain a very detailed understanding of a person's tendencies and behavior.

Watch 'Who are you, really? The puzzle of personality' presented by Brian Little on www.ted.com.

Dr. Brian Little is a personality psychologist. In this talk, you will hear him talk about the 'Big Five' and the OCEAN models of personality.

Use these to glean insights into your own personality and conscientiousness level. As we'll see, these will play an important role in how much effort you'll have to put into getting your prenatal health plan to stick.

How much do you identify with each of the 'Big 5' traits?

According the 'Big Five' theory of personality psychology, by looking at a person's unique combination of traits, you can gain a very detailed understanding of their behavior patterns. How much do you identify with each of the traits? Write a sentence or two regarding each of the 'Big Five' traits and how much they pertain to you in your journal.

1. Conscientiousness; I am self-disciplined, controlled, and strive for achievement.
2. Openness; I like to explore new experiences such as art, emotion, and ideas.
3. Agreeableness; I tend to get along well with others and keep them in mind.
4. Extraversion; I am highly sociable and like to be in the company of others.
5. Emotional range; I experience unpleasant emotions, such as anxiety, sadness, and anger on a regular basis.

STRATEGY 8: Make it a habit

You brush your teeth, yes? Twice a day? You just don't forget to do that because it's a habit. You're used to it, have embedded it into your routine, and have set, clear times for it, like before going to bed and immediately upon waking up in the morning.

Nobody roots for you or gives you candy, but you know that you did the right thing.

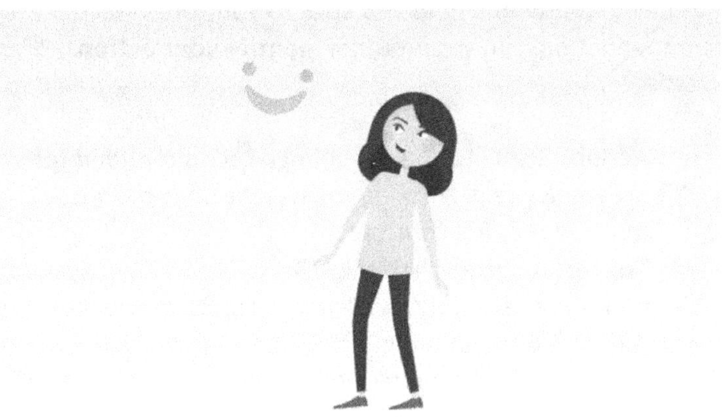

Approximately 40% of our actions during the day are habitual. The challenge is to create new habits when our health needs change, like during pregnancy.

What can you do to your chances of sticking to lifestyle changes like taking daily prenatals, changing your diet, and reducing your caffeine intake?

Research from the Health Behaviour Research Centre at the University College London shows that you can create new habits by connecting new actions to behaviors that are already automatic.

First, choose a small action that will become your new habit. Sticking to a small action will make it easier for you to succeed. Let's use the example of taking your prenatal vitamins.

Then, you need to attach it to a context, also called a trigger or a cue, which means an existing habit or routine. You might choose lunchtime, which you eat with your co-workers. Attach the habit to lunch so that from now on you take your pills at lunchtime. You can set a reminder on your phone or ask someone you eat with regularly to be on your case.

Finally, add a reward, which will build motivation by reinforcing the connection between the cue and the new behavior.

And you're set.

In summary, the newly formed habit should consist of:

- **An action** – Taking your vitamins, doing your prescribed exercises
- **A trigger or cue** – When you wake up, right before lunch, at 7 pm, etc.
- **A reward** – Complimenting yourself, having a piece of chocolate, or watching your favorite show

When you repeat this new behavior every day in the same context, it will soon become a habit. Habits that we create make life easier, point us in a desired direction, and are a great way to regulate our lives.

So, let's create a new health habit and make our prenatal plan stick.

What new habit would help you stick to your prenatal health recommendations? In your journal **identify your actions, triggers, and rewards:**

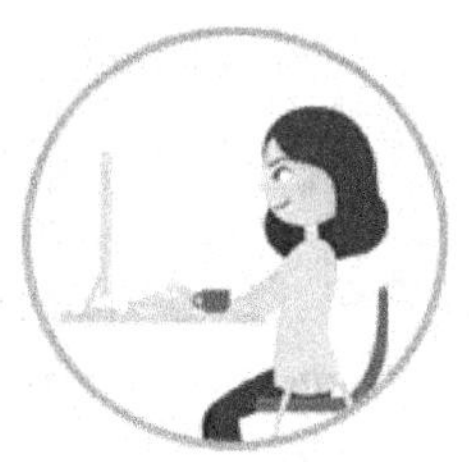

- **Action.** A small behavior change recommended for you during your pregnancy (e.g. *tracking my weight daily after doc says I gained too much in the first trimester*)
- **Trigger.** A current habit you have that can accommodate the action you choose for your new habit (e.g. *brushing my teeth in the morning*)
- **Reward.** Something internal, like a sense of accomplishment, or a small treat (*e.g. tell myself how wonderful I am for practicing healthy habits*)

TIPS

Tip 1: Check out the Habit Workshop course for a more comprehensive guide to building and sustaining habits.

Tip 2: To make the habit extra effective, set yourself up for success. For example – have a water bottle with you so it's easier to swallow the pill, have a snack in your bag in case you missed a meal but need to take your pill after eating, etc. Planning ahead will boost your adherence.

9 Good internal motivators for sticking to your pregnancy plan

Intrinsic motivation is the way to go if you want to establish a habit of your doctor's pregnancy requirements. Here are some great intrinsic motivators to help you feel rewarded for taking your folic acid, vitamins, or whatever else your doctor has advised.

1. I am keeping my body and my baby healthy.
2. As a mother, self-discipline is crucial. Better to already practice it now and stick to my plan when I need to.
3. Every pill, vitamin, and good dietary choice is a step in the right direction.
4. I love my baby, my body, and myself.
5. Every time I stick to my plan, I'm reminding myself how much I love my family. I'm giving to them by staying healthy.
6. I'm already starting to practice being a good role model for my children.

List some of your motivators:

7. ____

8. ____

9. ____

An external treat works just fine for my adherence

External rewards get a bad rap beyond the toddler years, and certainly in adulthood. But we're wondering, does it really make such a difference? The main thing is that you are sticking to your pregnancy plan, isn't it?

For:

1. A little regression into the toddler years never killed anyone. Straying from a doctor's orders during pregnancy may have. Just saying.
2. If it works, why make it harder for me? I'll just make sure I won't run out of my treats.
3. Who cares if a behavior is internally or externally motivated? A cookie is delicious. It will get me to take my pill. A "sense of satisfaction" will not. End of story.

How would an external treat help your adherence?

4. ____

Against:

1. It may work now, but it won't work in the long run.
2. Think of how hard it is to establish a habit. There's no way I'd give that all up for some measly chocolate chips.
3. I always do what the doctors order… and if they order intrinsic motivation now, then that's what I'll go for.

Or would the external treat hurt your ability to adhere to your pregnancy plan?

4. ____

The day I finally managed to adhere to my prenatal health plan

On that day you did everything right – and stuck to your prenatal plan – exactly the way you wanted to. How did you do it? How did it make you feel? Write about your experience in your journal.

Direct message us YOUR story @Buddy_N_Soul on Instagram and be anonymously featured for a chance to **win a Buddy&Soul three month free membership.**

Watch 'The Power of Habit' presented by Charles Duhigg at TEDxTeachersCollege on YouTube.

In the TED Talk presented by award-winning columnist and New York Times best-selling author Charles Duhigg, he explains how we can harness the power of habits.

As you listen to his talk, think about what health habits you want to create during your pregnancy, because, as Duhigg says, "you have the ability to change any habit in your life."

It's impossible to create a new habit when you're pregnant.

Which ancient philosopher said "you can't teach an old dog new tricks"? Did they mention that when the old dog is pregnant, nauseous, and in constant discomfort to boot, the very phrase "new tricks" ought to be unmentionable? I'm lucky if I can eat anything or move at all. Forget establishing new habits!

(Plus: Check out our Habit Workshop course for more.)

For:

1. With all the pressure of doing well for me and my baby I hardly have time or willpower to create new habits.
2. Everything is tough during pregnancy.
3. I'm way too focused on other things right now to start integrating new habits

What is one reason you struggle with creating these new habits?

4. ____

Against:

1. There's nothing like a new baby on the way to motivate me to make some changes in my habits.
2. Good habits will help make my pregnancy easier, not harder.
3. Everything is tough, so why not make some new habits while I'm at it?

Why is it beneficial for you to create these new habits?

4. ____

<u>STRATEGY 9: Make a pregnancy rule</u>

Being pregnant is more complex than it sounds from the outside. There are so many sudden changes that we're expected to make.

Whether you sacrifice a cigarette, a cup of coffee, or anything else that is not recommended for you and baby, you are being proactive and practicing a healthy pregnant lifestyle – kudos to you!

But, as we all know, it can be really difficult to make the right choice over and over again, day in, day out, for nine months straight.

Here is your chance to concretize your efforts to adhere to your health plan by making a rule that honors your efforts to maintain a healthy pregnancy.

It's a rule that will help you follow all the other rules, because there's an incentive built into it. Ideally, your rule should be positive and validate your efforts by rewarding you in some way. You can be as silly or as funny as you like — in fact, making it fun can remind you that pregnancy doesn't have to be such a serious time.

First, you'll need to choose a lifestyle change or another aspect of your prenatal health plan that you'd like to focus your rule around. Then, create a rule that will help you enjoy that experience. When it becomes a concrete rule as opposed to a mere suggestion, as Michael Raynor joked in his TED Talk about the Ten Commandments, it's easier for us to justify.

Here are some examples of pregnancy rules you may wish to adopt:

- For every item of clothing I grow out of, I buy a new one.
- If I took my prenatal vitamin, I get to eat my meal on the couch.
- For every cigarette that I didn't smoke, I pay myself a dollar.
- When I exercise like I should, I get extra TV time.

So, let's take some time to think about a rule that will make it more fun to stick to the rules.

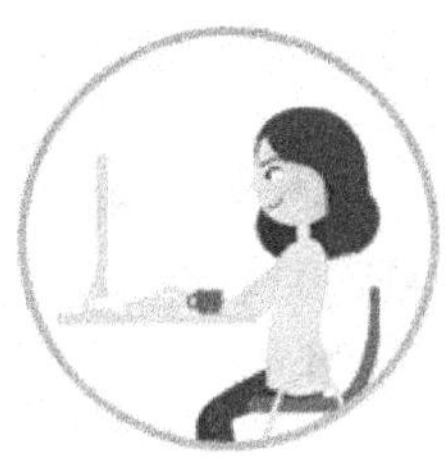

Create your own pregnancy rule that will help you stick to one of your health requirements and write it in your journal. You can use one of the examples we've discussed or come up with your own. Make sure to include your reward in the rule!

TIPS

Tip 1: Consider whether you might already be doing something to reward yourself for your efforts in adhering to your health plan and build on that.

Tip 2: You can broaden this exercise to include things like a positive outlook on life, singing to your baby every night before you go to bed, or sending your in-laws a weekly "bump" update.

You would happily take your prenatal meds daily if only:

Like any normal person, you want to do what's best for yourself and your baby. And, like any normal person, you're finding it tough to stick to the prenatal rules your doctor has given you. But you know you would gladly adhere to properly taking your folic acid and any other pregnancy meds if only…

1. You were able to find enough time to breathe during the course of the day.
2. The simple act of introducing it into your mouth didn't make you regurgitate your breakfast (read: single corn flake).
3. Someone came up with an invention to counter pregnancy brain and you could actually remember things.
4. It didn't make you feel like you had some kind of disease that required medicating.
5. You felt that it was something you really needed to do.

What would help you take your prenatal meds?

6. ____

7. ____

8. ____

Fun rules to help you ace your prenatal adherence

Whoever says pregnancy is a serious time has got it all wrong. Here are some fun ideas for pregnancy rules that will put a smile on your face while helping you stick to your pregnancy plan. Perhaps they'll even inspire you to create some of your own.

1. Every time I pass up a social drink, I go home and have a Madonna dance party!
2. Every prenatal vitamin is preceded by me getting into victory pose and roaring like a lion.
3. Prenatal vitamins are to be taken while blindfolded. I have my partner hand me a mini jelly bean or a vitamin.
4. Every time I take a pill or vitamin, my partner has to do a push-up.
5. For every willpower win, I call my best friend for voracious applause.

Can you think of any fun rules that will help you to adhere to your pregnancy plan?

6. ____

7. ____

8. ____

(Plus: Check out our Willpower 101 course for more.)

The pregnancy rule that hugely impacted my health

When you create a pregnancy rule, you eliminate half the battle, as there is no longer any need to negotiate with yourself. What was your rule and how did it help improve your health? Reflect on your experience in your journal.

Direct message us YOUR story @Buddy_N_Soul on Instagram and be anonymously featured for a chance to **win a Buddy&Soul three month free membership.**

Have you heard of the saying "Rules are meant to be broken?"

In this TED talk, Michael Raynor tells us that the exact opposite is true – rules were made to be followed, especially when we are tempted to break them.

Watch 'Three Rules for Success' presented by Michael Raynor at TEDxUniversityofNevada on YouTube.

As you watch this insightful clip, think about what rules do for you and how they can help you live according to your values.

Sticking to the rules is impossible when you're pregnant

If you have a hard time following rules at the best of times, it's probably safe to assume your struggle is magnified tenfold during pregnancy. And yet, precisely when it's become that much more challenging – bam! They hit you with a whole new set of rules relating to diet, lifestyle, meds, and prenatal health. They've gotta be kidding!

For:

1. Pregnancy is so unpredictable. How can I possibly follow rules when everything is changing all the time?
2. Pregnancy is a time where you are meant to *break* the rules. Like eating pickles and ice cream together or non-stop Netflix cryathons.
3. Now's my chance to have a good time before I have to become a rule-keeping mommy.

Why do you find it challenging to stick to the rules of your pregnancy plan?

4. ____

Against:

1. Pregnancy is *the* time to follow the rules. Every little bit counts toward a healthy baby.
2. With a little help and support from doctors, family, and friends there's no reason why I can't succeed at sticking to my pregnancy plan.
3. Knowing that pregnancy is only for a set period of time and that there's an end in sight makes it easier for me to stick to things. I know that at the end of these 9 months I can simply re-evaluate.

Why is it important for you to stick to these pregnancy plan rules?

4. ____

STRATEGY 10: Celebrate your self-control

When you realize that you've accomplished something big by sticking to your prenatal health plan, you owe it to yourself to take that pat on the back!

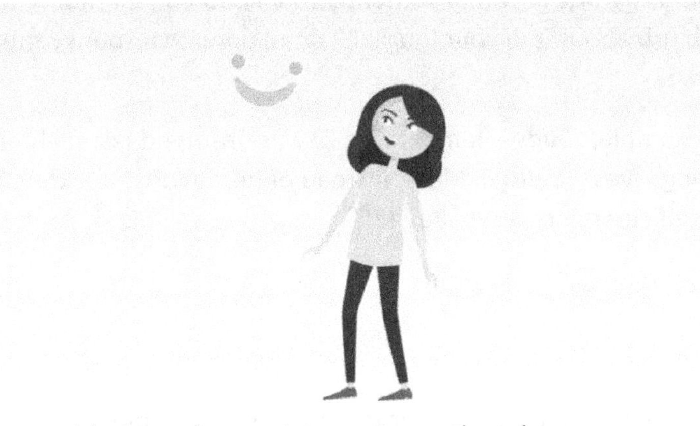

We're talking about every small step that you took towards success – choosing a restaurant that wouldn't tempt with the sushi menu, packing your vitamins and folic acid for the babymoon to Atlantic City, not skipping last week's doctor's appointment even though you could have slept all day, drinking a glass of water because it's good for you, even though it couldn't be less appealing.

Each step is worth celebrating, no matter how small, because it leads you in the right direction and builds your willpower muscle.

And if you've experienced setbacks and aren't entirely following your doctor's guidelines yet?

As the saying goes 'Rome wasn't built in a day.' If you're here, learning from this book, it shows that you care and that in itself is a success.

Take the time to review and reflect on your accomplishments, and be encouraged that you can do it.

Ready? Set? Let's go!

EXERCISE

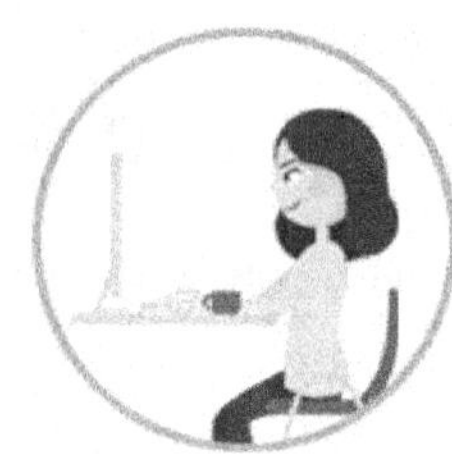

Action: **Imagine a tabloid magazine featuring you on their front page, celebrating one accomplishment you've had while reading this book.** Write the blurb about it in your journal, jazzed up with a spunky tabloid alias of course.

For example, "Super-Bump Rayna Z. was observed last night in the hippest bar in town sipping – yes – a Virgin Mary, instead of her favorite cocktail. We appreciate the irony, and the self-restraint. Bravo, Rayna!"

TIPS

Tip 1: Look back through your journal to remind yourself of some of your accomplishments (pregnancy brain, we hear ya!).

Tip 2: For extra fun, share your story with the Buddy and Soul community! Tag us on Instagram and Twitter @Buddy_N_Soul, using the #BuddynSoulExpecting. By sharing with us on social media, not only can you help others with their personal journeys, you can read about those facing similar challenges.

Bragging won't improve my prenatal health!

It's always nice to give myself a pat on the back or a high five. But will it impact how well I adhere to my doctor's prenatal plan? I doubt it!

For:

1. Bragging is bragging. It's just words. It's not connected at all to behavior.
2. I usually brag about things I'm not actually doing...it draws attention away from that embarrassing fact.
3. Sure, bragging *feels* great, but it usually stops there.

Add your own:

4. ____

Against:

1. Bragging brings to doing more, so of course it helps!
2. When I brag about something, I'm suddenly accountable and have to follow through. And if I don't, I'll have 950 disappointed social media followers to answer to!
3. I'll try anything that can help me stick to my pregnancy plan. Besides, a little bragging seems harmless.

Add your own:

4. ____

What prenatal health goals are you celebrating today?

Human nature is such that we tend to remember the negative and forget the positive. For that reason, it's extra important to make a concerted effort to dwell on your accomplishments, no matter how small. So, what gains have you made with properly adhering to your prenatal health regimen and requirements? Because it's time to celebrate!

1. Every cup of coffee I skipped.
2. Each time I chose water over wine.
3. Skipping the raw fish in my sushi.
4. Cooked eggs over runny ones.
5. Going to the doctor regularly, as required.
6. Not binging on junk food.
7. Taking the stairs instead of the elevator.
8. Getting a good night's sleep instead of going out.
9. Tossing my cigarettes and not buying replacements.
10. Taking my prenatal vitamins every single (friggin') day.

What else are you celebrating?

11. ____

12. ____

13. ____

When you started this book, you didn't know what you might accomplish. Here you are at the finish line, and you've made it through! Take five minutes to write about your biggest success in your journal.

Direct message us YOUR greatest accomplishments @Buddy_N_Soul on Instagram and be anonymously featured for a chance to **win a Buddy&Soul three month free membership.**

DRIVING THE MESSAGE HOME

You are almost at the end of the Sticking to Your Pregnancy Plan book where we'll finally take a look back at your accomplishments and celebrate our successes.

But before we do that, let's finish with a powerful TED talk by John Wooden, head coach of the UCLA basketball team. You'll hear his definition of success and how it formed his career and influenced the players on his team.

Watch 'The Difference Between Winning and Succeeding' presented by John Wooden on YouTube.

Use it to boost your motivation for continued, future success, even once you finish this book!

What's your definition of success this pregnancy?

Success is definitely something that's in the eye of the beholder. So, what is your own personal definition of success this pregnancy? Remember that success is not only about the big things. The little things count too!

1. Getting out of bed every morning and getting all my basic responsibilities done.
2. Taking my vitamins on a regular basis.
3. Not missing a prenatal appointment.
4. Getting the help I've needed. And boy have I needed a lot of it!
5. Staying away from those things that have pregnancy warnings on them, like cigarettes and alcohol.
6. Cutting myself some slack. Being pregnant is really hard!

List more of your successes:

7. ____

8. ____

9. ____

What got you to stick to your prenatal health plan?

Now that you've completed the Sticking to Your Pregnancy Plan course, you know what helped you improve your adherence and what didn't. Which of the following worked best for you?

1. Setting an alarm.
2. Having a support buddy.
3. A medication app.
4. Preplanning.
5. Better educating myself.
6. Talking to my OB/GYN and medical team.

Was there anything else that helped you?

7. ____

8. ____

9. ____

WHERE DO WE GO FROM HERE?

You've finished the Sticking to Your Pregnancy Plan book, but you haven't finished the journey. It doesn't end, it just gets better. Revisit this book, carry its ideas with you. Check out BuddynSoul.com and the rest of our books for all we have to offer. Spread the word. And change your life for good.

You've finished the Sticking to Your Pregnancy Plan book, but you haven't finished the journey. It doesn't end, it just gets better. Revisit this book, carry its ideas with you. Check out BuddynSoul.com and the rest of our books for all we have to offer. Spread the word. And change your life for good.

Loving Your Pregnant Body

Pregnancy can feel like an alien invasion right inside your body! If you're finding it challenging to come to terms with some of the changes your body is going through, welcome to the club. In this book, you'll find helpful, research-based actions you can take to keep your self-esteem up and your unfounded expectations down this pregnancy, no matter what changes your body is going through.

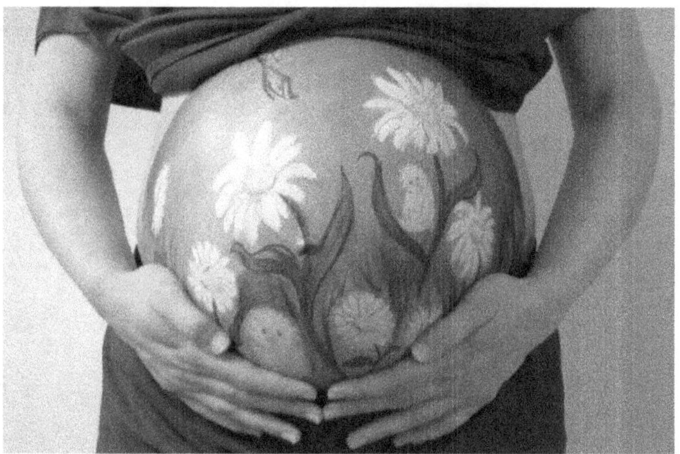

<u>Goals you can achieve by reading 'Loving your Pregnant Body':</u>

1. Accept your body regardless of its changes.
2. Let go of critical thoughts, fears, and unrealistic expectations around your pregnant body.
3. Appreciate the changes in your body as a part of the miracle of creating a new life

Relationship Saver During Pregnancy

Pregnancy can put a strain on even the best relationships. That's why it's so important to preemptively support your relationship now, so your new family can be built on rock-solid foundations. Keeping in mind your needs, your partner's needs, and the needs of your relationship, this course will give you the know-how to strengthen your connection during pregnancy and beyond.

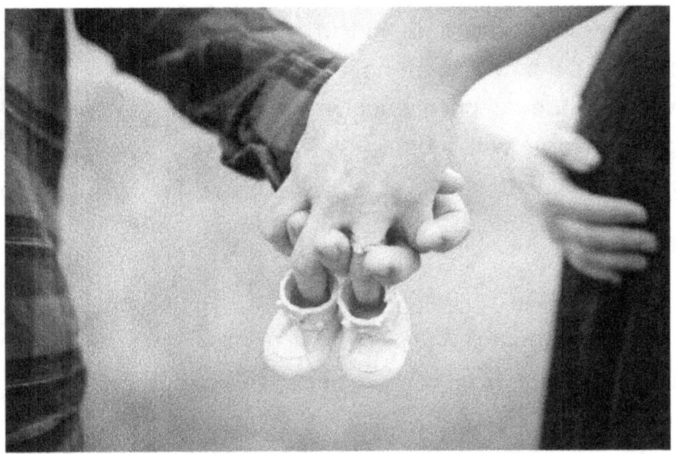

<u>Goals you can achieve by reading 'Relationship Saver During Pregnancy'</u>:

1. Identify your needs – both as two individuals and as a pair – as you navigate this pregnancy.
2. Strengthen your communication and build your connection with your partner.
3. Take responsibility for improving your relationship during pregnancy and beyond.

Acing the Fourth Trimester

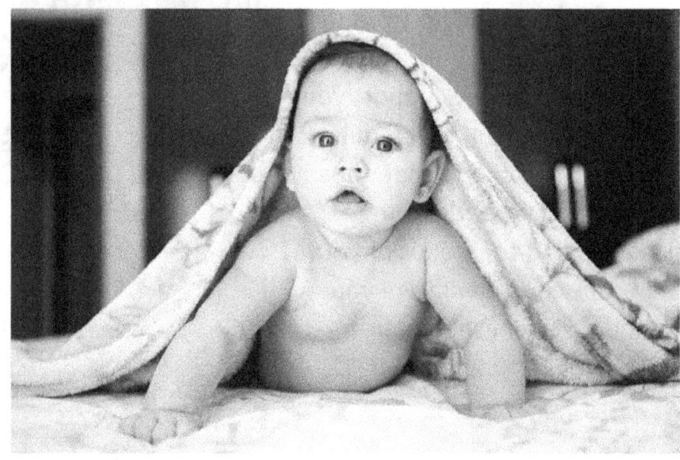

It is a universally acknowledged truth that much like a Jane Austen novel ends with a wedding, once you give birth and go home with a baby you end up at home with a new baby.

And experience pure bliss.

Now, back to reality. Considering that you're still hormonal and bleeding, possibly recovering from surgery or stitching, and your baby basically is a fetus with a vocal range that suddenly carries, it's not surprising that the first three months after birth are referred to as the "fourth trimester." Unfortunately, the books, websites, and apps seem to stop after three; those that *do* discuss the first year, focus almost solely on the newborn. Once the baby's out you're no longer a part of the pregnancy community, but you're not quite a part of the parenting fold, either. And you're certainly not back to your old self – with sleep, habits, stress, anything and everything that a tiny creature can and will throw off (but aren't they cute?).

That's where we come in. Join us to learn how to juggle this time of emotional ups and downs, of changing relationships, habits, and priorities. No matter how your baby came into the world, you're indisputably handling a lot more than you used to. We'll provide you with the tools you need to ace the fourth trimester, making your postnatal adjustment smoother, easier, and more enjoyable.

<u>Goals you can achieve by reading 'Acing the Fourth Trimester':</u>

1. Process your birth experience, whether it was positive, negative, or somewhere in the middle,
2. Learn strategies to help ease the difficult parts of your fourth trimester,
3. Help you create a post-birth roadmap to get you back to you.

WANT TO LEARN MORE? CHECK THESE OUT!

MOVIES

What to Expect When You're Expecting (2012)

Inspired by the perennial bestseller, What to Expect When You're Expecting is a hilarious and heartfelt comedy about five couples whose intertwined lives are turned upside down by the challenges of impending parenthood.

Watch and enjoy how each woman manages the gifts and challenges of pregnancy and motherhood, including the struggle of feeling good in her pregnant body.

40 Weeks (2014)

40 Weeks is the first unscripted documentary film to offer an intimate window into the week-by-week journey of pregnant women across the country.

40 Weeks explores the emotional and physical changes of pregnancy, the hopes and fears, and the confusing and often difficult choices that can be presented during this time.

MORE VIDEOS

Picturing pregnancy: Meredith Nash at TEDxHobart

In 2011, Meredith Nash asked a question that no other sociologist had asked before: How would women document their experiences of pregnancy if they were given a camera?

She gave pregnant Tasmanian women digital cameras and asked them to photograph whatever they felt best captured their lives and experiences. Two years and 2000 photographs later, she explains why these pictures invite new possibilities for thinking about pregnancy and body image.

(Plus: Check out our Loving Your Pregnant Body course 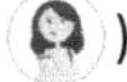)

You're Talking to Me? Ensuring patient comprehension, motivation and personalization

Watch Buddy&Soul's co-founder Dr. Talya Miron-Shatz speak about how to improve your medical compliance by improving your participation in your own medical care plan. Talya discusses the importance of enabling patients to take a more active role in their healthcare decisions.

Learn what factors can help you assert yourself when making decisions about your prenatal plan.

RECOMMENDED APPS

MyMed Schedule

This free app reminds you when to take your medications with email and/or text notifications.

A great app for you if you're having trouble remembering to take your prenatal vitamins, iron, folic acid, or any other prescribed daily meds.

MommyMeds - Pregnancy Safety Guide

MommyMeds mobile app is the premier health & safety app for all pregnant and breastfeeding mothers. Ensure your baby's safety while using prescription and over-the-counter medication.

Just search or scan the barcodes of thousands of medications and receive immediate, easy-to-understand information on drug safety and ingredients.

If the fine print about your medication isn't clear, use this app to make sure it's safe for you.

Mom.life — Pregnancy tracker and support for moms

This is an app for moms. It's real life, not the highlight reel. Be authentic, candid and real in this live moderated social community of moms from pregnancy, baby stages and beyond. No mom shaming allowed!

Find useful advice for staying on track before, during and after your pregnancy. Maintain a healthy pregnancy diet through tips and recommended pregnancy food trackers from moms like you.

Learn about pregnancy fitness - pregnancy yoga, safe pregnancy exercise and postpartum workout ideas. Includes a chat and community feature.

If you are looking for support from other pregnant moms, this app is a great way to do that without getting off the couch!

BOOKS

Habit Stacking: 127 Small Changes to Improve Your Health, Wealth, and Happiness (Most are Five Minutes or Less) by S.J. Scott

Imagine what life would be like if you started every morning with small actions that created a chain reaction of positive benefits throughout your life. You eat a healthy breakfast, have a great conversation with your loved ones, and then begin your workday focusing on the important tasks. Then, throughout the day, you foster habits that support your goals. You'd probably feel more fulfilled, get more accomplished, and have a better direction for your career.

And all this can be done when you follow a strategy known as "Habit Stacking" as S.J. Scott describes in this book.

If you are feeling drained by your pregnancy, you'll find some helpful tips in this book to help you maintain the habits that are most important to you.

(Plus: Check out our Habit Workshop course 🧑 for more.)

How to Take Charge of Your Health: Handbook to Navigate Today's Medical Visits by Susan Cooper

This book by Susan Cooper gives you tips for making the most of your doctor visits, as long as you are of sound enough mind and body to ask questions and make your wishes known. Advice about what to do and where to go in a medical emergency are an extra bonus.

If you are concerned about the medical care you are receiving during your pregnancy, this is an important read.

The Patient from Hell: How I Worked with my Doctors to Get the Best of Modern Medicine and How You Can Too by Stephen H. Schneider and Janica Lane

A personal account of how one patient – an experienced doctor himself – conducted in-depth research about his medical condition and worked with (and sometimes against) the doctors treating him to modify his treatment plan.

The Patient from Hell by Stephen H. Schneider and Janica Lane is a good book to read if you need encouragement to advocate for your medical care.

Perfect for the gal who intends to be actively involved in her pregnancy-related medical choices.

Vital Conversations: Improving Communication between Doctors and Patients by Dennis Rosen

Vital Conversations by Dennis Rosen seeks to prove that excellent communication between doctors and patients has a direct impact on the quality of treatment and final prognosis of patients.

Use this book as a guide to help you get the best treatment possible from your medical care providers.

If you are determined to get the best prenatal care, reading this book will help you achieve your goals.

GADGETS AND PRODUCTS

<u>Medcenter Talking Alarm Clock And Medication Reminder</u>

This helpful talking alarm clock can remind you to take your medication up to 4 times daily. It features a friendly female voice that can be programmed with additional pleasant messages, such as good morning. It is battery operated, and small enough to carry around with you.

Perfect for those of us who are memory-challenged while pregnant and need an extra reminder to keep up with their pregnancy supplements and vitamins.

<u>MedCenter 31-Day Pill Organizer</u>

Do you have trouble organizing your vitamins, or remembering whether you took your pills? This 31-day pill organizer has 31 separate boxes to help you pre-organize your pills by the month.

It has easy-to-open lids that allow for easy access and a convenient color-coding system that shows when a daily dose is complete.

This organizer will help you remember to take your prenatal vitamins and whatever else the doctor ordered during your pregnancy.